Also by Dr. Stenbeck

Available from the usual on-line source

Books
Healing Yourself -- The Holistic Approach
    [An introduction to Holistic Self-healing.]

Heal Yourself Right Now!
    [The Seven Priority Organ Levels for
    effective Nutritional/Holistic Treatment of
    all organs.]

The 22 Unique Body Types
    (for Health and Weight Loss)

Q & A to Identify Your Body Type (Booklet)
    [Individual Type booklets are also available

Booklets
(Step-by-step instructions on healing yourself)

    #1 Start Healing with Positive Thinking
    #2 Mastering Positive Feelings for Health!
    #3 Spiritual Balance and Your Healing

The Barotic Body Type

Representing one of the 22 Body Types first described by Victor Rocine around 1900

The Robin Williams, 'Mrs. Doubtfire' Celebrity Body Type

For Kaye,
there at the beginning with Doc Severn,
and for Liberty,
continuing the holistic healing journey...

Disclaimer

———

About the Author

Educated in New Zealand and in the U.S.A., Dr. Stenbeck attained B.Sc. (NZ), M.S., and D.C. degrees. His holistic healing methods have been profiled in magazines (Esquire, McLean's, Playgirl, the Atlanta Constitution), and on TV in the USA and in Canada. He was the main contributor to the Warner Book, _The Eye/Body Connection_ by Jessica Maxwell that focused on the holistic healing relationships between the iris structure and organ genetics.

In the 1970-80's he was elected Fellow, Royal Society of Health, London; Fellow, American Association of Chemists; Member, American Association of Clinical Chemists; and Affiliate, Royal Society of Medicine, London. He studied naturopathy and Body Types with Dr. Bernard Jensen and Dr. Clifford Severn, and has practiced in medical partnerships where patients received the joint benefits of medical and holistic healing.

He is a member of Self-Realization Fellowship. To receive advice on any health issue from a holistic viewpoint, or to receive help with your body type, see his web site: *DrStenbeck.net*

———

Contents

* * *

The Barotic Body Type and Food Guide

Appendix

* * *

The 22 Body Types:
Celebrity Examples

This Booklet contains the Barotic type. See
The 22 Unique Body Types for all type
descriptions.]

Thin Types

Atrophic *Woody Allen / Audrey Hepburn*
Stan Laurel / Calista Flockheart

Exesthesic *Cher / Sarah Jessica Parker*
(Female type only)

Marasmic *President Obama / Princess Diana*
James Stewart / Kate Blanchard

Neurogenic *J.K. Simmons / Joan Rivers*
Jon Cryer / Marin Hinle

Pathoferic *(No celebrity males)*
Blythe Danner / Gwyneth Paltrow

Sillevitic *David Bowie / Shirley MacLaine*
Rod Stewart / Carol Channing

Muscle Types

Calciferic	Michael Jordan / Angelica Huston Abrahma Lincoln / Grace Jones
Carbogenic	George Clooney / Lady Gaga Pres. G. Bush, Jr., Meg Ryan
Desmogenic	Marlon Brando / Loni Anderson Daniel Craig / Tina Turner
Eldic	Ross Perot / Hillary Clinton Peter Falk / Sigourney Weaver
Myogenic	Pres. Bill Clinton / Sharon Stone Pres. John Kennedy / Julia Roberts
Nervimotive	Frank Sinatra / Elizabeth Taylor Mark Wahlberg / Natalie Wood
Nitropheric	Ben Affleck / Ava Gardner Kirk Douglas / Kate Winslet
Pallinomic	Pres. Donald Trump / Attorney General Janet Reno Bill O'Reilly (Fox) / Jane Russell

Fat Types

Barotic   *Robin Williams / 'Mrs.Doubtfire'*
              Elton John / William Conrad

Carboferic *Bill Murray / Roseanne*
              Billy Gardell / Melissa McCarthy

Hydripheric *John Goodman / Shelly Winters*
              Wayne Knight / Jennifer Holliday

Isogenic   *Einstein / Oprah Winfrey*
              Phillip S .Hoffman / Queen Victoria

Lipopheric *Rush Limbaugh / Rosie O'Donnell*
              Chris Christie / Camryn Manheim

Oxypheric   *Winston Churchill / Orsen Welles*
              Ella Fitzgerald / Gerry Spence

Pargenic   *Burt Reynolds / Katey Segal*
              Ron Perlman / Kirstey Alley

<u>*Succinct Quote on Human Types*</u>

From Victor Rocine, who first described discrete body types around 1900.

"A type is an order of people that differentiates and distinguishes itself by a general and similar form, brain-formation, chemistry, structure, build, immunity, tendencies, predisposition, resemblance, skin-pigment, and type characteristics based on observation and analogy.

"Or, in other words, people of a given type are similar physically and like-minded as if they were brothers and sisters—that is what type means.

"Everything in nature is made according to plan. Man only discovers that plan and gives it a name. The zoologist has not made the animals—he has only described the plan adopted by the wonderful Creator, and named the classes, sub-classes, etc.

"How important type research will be to humanity, time alone will make known."

———

Prologue

The esteemed scientist J. J. Berzelius, discoverer of several chemical elements, inspired Victor Rocine to research body types and to investigate the correlation between types and their diseases. Around 1890-1910, Rocine privately published his original findings on the mineral basis of different body types, and this present book exists because of his brilliant insights.

For many years, I studied with Dr. Clifford Severn who had been a personal student of Victor Rocine on body types, naturopathy, herbology, iris analysis, diet, and nutritional healing methods. He had a successful career as a lecturer and healer, and was one of those rare athletes with complete muscle control over his body. I saw him under a spotlight at 85 years of age, contracting and rippling every individual muscle in his perfectly developed body. Field-Marshal Jan Smuts, the WWII South African Prime Minister, devoted a full chapter of his autobiography to how Severn's healing methods had saved his life. In the 1950's, *Life* magazine did a four-page spread on Severn and his family. Fame he had.

Another Rocine student I studied with, Dr. Bernard Jensen wrote of Rocine's body type research and nutritional methods in his privately published, *The Chemistry of Man*.

This book is deeply rooted in Rocine's original work, and with that of Herbert Shelton, M.D., Ph.D. (at Harvard University in the 1930's). I integrated their research with newer dietary and nervous system data along with celebrity examples of each type, hopefully, making this material easier to digest and more entertaining for the reader.

Gayelord Hauser, another Rocine student I knew, was a celebrated health book author. He wrote a popular book on Rocine's types in the 1940's, *Types and Temperaments;* reputedly, he also introduced yogurt to the western world.

This book exists because of Rocine's creative brilliance and original discoveries in natural healing.

▶ *Rocine: "The soul creates the body type."*

Rocine taught that the soul chooses a body type and brain to live in, thus presenting different experiences and life lessons to master. Why were *you* born the way you are?

That is something to think about, especially if it is true! What would your soul purpose be to live in a particular body type. I provide some thoughts on this issue in each type description and try to assess from my experience with your type the particular lessons of life presented therein.

Rocine was as brilliant in his way as an Abraham Lincoln, Michael Jordan, Michael Phelps, Tony Robbins, or a Daniel Day Lewis—all *calciferic* types—rare, leaders, innovative, brilliant, and highly intelligent in their different fields of endeavor.

Celebrity examples exist for most types, not a duplicate of you, but someone who has your essence in their body-mind individuality. Knowing your type allows you to become a better you!

The celebrity examples provide further help in identifying your body type.

▶ *Rocine's classic findings are the backbone of this book. Integrated with Sheldon's research and with other dietary and food issues including mental, emotional, and spiritual attributes,*

Many people take nutritional supplements and try different diets without a doctor's advice. If this is your choice, use common sense, listen to body responses, and discontinue any allergic reactions to foods or nutritional substances.

———

The Barotic Body Type

"*You may also have a physical or psychological feature not representative of your type such as height, weight, appearance, talent, weakness, strength, etc., due to biochemical errors, environmental influences, racial or cultural differences, and congenital or genetic issues. Nevertheless, the type identification of the average person is usually clear.*"

—*Victor Rocine*

Barotic Type
Celebrity Examples

If you think this is your type, be sure to look at **on-line photographs** *of these examples. Look for general similarities to yourself. Note that sub-types cause the differences in appearance between members of the same type. You are a relatively rare type, with few males and no representative female examples.*

————

ACTING/TV

Robin Williams (His genius is apparent!
    You may be two or three times heavier
    than him.)

'Mrs. Doubtfire' (In this movie, Robin
    Williams provides an idea of how this
    lady may look. Check her out!)

William Conrad ("Jake and the Fat Man";
    "Cannon" TV series)

Sebastian Cabot
Burl Ives
[Most of us have seen this type on TV.]

ARTS & MUSIC

Peter Jackson (director "Lord of the
Rings")
Elton John

*[Note: I personally knew several members of
this type, which contributed to my understanding of
the type. My best childhood friend was this type,
an esteemed photographer.*

Read the types, and if still confused you
may choose to use the personal request for
type identification from my web site:
DrStenbeck.net

——————

Barotic Type Questionnaire

These questions describe the generic type, and not specifically you! If any question ever applied to you, then choose the True answer!

For Question 1 only:

A = True	*B = Maybe*	*C = Untrue*
15 points	*7 points*	*1 point*

1. Physically identify with celebrity example ____

Then..

A = True	*B = Maybe*	*C = Untrue*
5 points	*3 points*	*1 point*

---

2. Height is close to:
   Males: 5'5-6'8   Females: 5'5-6'2   ____
3. Usual weight is close to:
   Males: 185-330+   Females: 165-230+   ____
4. Large and bony, broad body with a
   flat front and back (if not heavy)   ____
5. Masculine body (both sexes)   ____
6. Highly practical, honest, and ethical   ____
7. Peaceful, plain, innocent looking   ____
8. Good hair growth, later in life may
   bald from back-head forwards;
   often enjoy a full-beard   ____
9. Patience, acceptance, passivity, and
   non-aggression are strong traits   ____
10. Wide lips, mouth; lower lip is often flat____

11. Broad face, no cheek indentations;
    wide cheek-bones; wide jaws _____
12. Highly humane and caring of others _____
13. White teeth, average-sized or smaller _____
14. Mostly non-addictive personality
    (may over-indulge in gourmet foods
    and alcohol) _____
15. Love to serve mankind and others _____
16. Mind 'latent' with potential _____
17. Speak the truth plainly; do not defer
    to what others need to hear _____
18. Passionate, moral, ethical _____
19. Great in emergencies: able to step
    forward and take charge _____
20. Generally non-judgmental of others _____
21. Honest and reliable _____
22. Strong will-power when motivated! _____
23. Weak decisiveness and motivation _____
24. Academic plodders, hard to take
    exams, slow decision making _____
25. Appear timid (but are brave as lions
    when necessary) _____
26. Make life-long friends; are warm, loyal
    sociable, interested, communicative _____
27. Humility and humanity is genuine _____
28. Use love and understanding to forgive _____
29. Are strict disciplinarians _____
30. Strong self-depreciating tendency _____
31. Philosophers, love God, the universe;
    are naturalists, may -be metaphysical _____
32. Have abundant faith, hope, courage _____

33. Suppress and have difficulty expressing deep feelings (love, hate, etc.) _____
34. Inappropriate trust of people _____
35. If severely wronged by someone, that person can then do nothing right _____
36. Shy and reticent until aroused _____
37. Have intense dislikes _____
38. 'Slow to ripen'; need to feel appreciated for talents _____
39. Gentle, peaceful, inoffensive _____
40. Excellent ability to socialize, converse with anyone _____
41. Almost impossible to kill or go to war (unlike other fat types) _____
42. Are wise, make excellent judges _____
43. Sexual drive medium or sluggish, and rarely a priority _____
44. Respect people who work for a living; have little time for the homeless _____
45. Dislike laziness _____
46. Disapprove strongly of cruelty _____
47. Need to be left alone on the job; supervise self and others well _____
48. Need time alone within a relationship _____
49. Love outdoor activities _____
50. Highly practical _____
51. Are prized employees for honesty and work-ethic _____
52. Usually not highly educated _____
53. Dislike lazy people, vanity, crime, ugliness, and chaos _____
54. Are health-minded _____

55. Love cooking, home-making, etc. _____
56. Loyal, law abiding, and hard working _____
57. Slow in committing to loving someone _____
58. Not athletic unless young; may be very
    good at swimming, wrestling, football _____
59. Able to apply principles, laws, facts,
    and theories _____

▶ *The type questionnaire pinpoints the major features of that type: if the celebrity examples are unhelpful, you may be an unusual variant (in which case ignore the celebrity issue and give yourself 7 points on Question 1)*

Scoring

For question #1:

A response: give 15 points = _____
B response: give 7 points = _____
C response: give 1 points = _____

For questions #2—59:

A response: give 5 points = _____
B response: give 3 points = _____
C response: give 1 point = _____

Total of the above points = _____

Interpretation

140—260: PROBABLY Barotic type
70—139: POSSIBLY Barotic type
<70: NOT Barotic type

The Barotic Type

Rocine: "Barotic means heavy in 'body, mind, and thoughts'. You utilize more <u>calcium and carbon</u> making you large, strong, friendly, and fat." You are intelligent, intellectual, personable, humble, friendly, sociable, plain-speaking, and peace-loving.

————

Y ou are mostly medium-tall, or tall, and when younger may be moderate-sized (like Robin Williams); you always fight the battle of the bulge. Typically, you are larger and look like the prior TV stars William Conrad and Sebastian Cabot.

▶ *Rocine: "You are like an eagle with a broken wing, a giant in chains, a mighty slumbering soul."*
[High praise indeed from the type master!]

You are personable, calm, humble, friendly, sociable, plain-speaking, and peace-loving. You are predominantly a male type with few female examples. Robin Williams in drag provides a valuable glimpse of the female appearance! You are like a sleeping bear: when aroused you act with force, determination, and brilliance; a diamond in the rough. Many German, Swede, Scotch, and Russians are this type.

▶ *You are never egocentric—very different to most other endomorphs!*

––––––

Physical Similarity to Other Types

The *carboferic* type (John Arnold, Roseanne Barr) is somewhat similar but more humorous, and less approachable.

The *lipopheric* type (Jackie Gleason, Ricki Lake) is also large, more intellectual and talkative, and usually less philosophical.

The *oxypheric* type (Winston Churchill, Ella Fitzgerald) is more naturally friendly and expressive, with a larger head and jaw.

––––––

Average Height and Weight

| Males: | 5'5-6'8 | 185-330+ pounds |
| Females: | 5'5-6'2 | 165-230+ pounds |

You already know something about this type from their public persona and appearance, whether from seeing them yourself or from the celebrity examples. Blend such insights with the type descriptions and the types of your family and friends to discern their presence in your midst!

———

Barotic Type Description

The type description represents how you appear in everyday society. You may have a sub-type that alters parts of this description.

Think of the celebrity examples as you read the descriptions. You have a large build, bony, and powerful in bones, joints, membranes, and muscles. Your broadness is a marked feature: the body is long and broad with a flat front and back appearing like a rectangle (which distorts as you add a large abdomen). You live in a genetically-ordained fat body: you can lose weight, and most of you have the necessary discipline to achieve it.

▶ *I have met only a few female barotics, but have seen many in Europe. She has a masculine look and nature, and is very practical (like the pallinomic lady). See Robin in the 'Mrs. Doubtfire'..*

Head — A long head with a large backhead is usual, somewhat like the *oxypheric*. Your forehead usually shows numerous so-called 'humanitarian' lines that reflect who you are: a friend to many. One *barotic* I know communicated regularly by mail (before e-mail) with scores of friends around the world. You are a friend to many.

Hair — The male body is often very hairy. Your hair is usually brown or dark; hair growth is excellent, and you often have a full-beard (rarer in other fat types); a slight balding occurs at the back-head with aging.

Eyes — Large, full, pleasant, and inviting eyes are usual; the eyesight is strong.

Ears — Your ears are large, thick, and positioned close to the head.

Nose — A broad nose is usual.

Face — Your face is broad without cheek indentations, wide from cheekbone to cheekbone; heavy, wide jaws.

▶ *Rocine: "You have a vase-shaped face, wide in the central portion, narrower at the temples (denoting low ego-strength, opposite to the desmogenic, lipopheric, and oxypheric wide temples)."*

Mouth, Lips and Voice — A wide mouth and lips are common, with a larger flat lower lip. Your voice is masculine, low-pitched, warm, and inviting.

Teeth — Your teeth are white, usually small or average sized.

Skin — Usually, you have a red 'ruddy' thick skin.

Neck — The neck is thick and fleshy.

Muscles — Although large and fat, your muscles are strong; your active fat metabolism precludes most athletics, but when younger you may be a wrestler, swimmer, or weight-lifter.

Chest — You have a large barrel-like chest, with a medium-sized or large bust.

Back and Shoulders — Your back is strong and broad.

Hips and Abdomen — The abdomen remains large and flat until you acquire fat; your hips are wide and ideal for childbirth; the waist is wide, strong, and high on the body.

Arms and Legs — Your extremities are heavy, long, and powerful; you have a slow, ponderous, shambling walk (but are able to move quickly). The wrists are large, fleshy and strong, the fingers long and graceful, your gestures purposeful and controlled.

▶ *The females have powerful limbs and bodies with a masculine build.*

Joints — Your bones and joints are strong and powerful, with an arthritis tendency (due to dietary inadequacies).

———

Barotic Personality Traits

If you are this type many, but not all, of the following characteristics are present—you may have overcome or moderated the negatives, but recognize that you once had several of them.

You may show any of the following traits.
- Dislike loud noises
- Great love of children

- Speak your truth plainly
- Not hurried or upset easily
- Are brave if forced to fight
- Talking heart-to-heart is your forte
- Are inoffensive, will not harm others
- Passionate with a wry sense of humor
- Are highly humane, born to be pacifists
- Truth, ethics and morality motivate you
- Have pragmatism, practicality, usefulness

▶ *Hallmarks of your personality are patience, gentleness, acceptance, passivity, and non-belligerence.*

- Cannot kill or go to war (unlike most fat types)
- Do not defer to what people want to hear from you
- Great in emergencies: will step forward and take charge
- Mind latent and pregnant with potential, but often undeveloped
- Academic plodders, slow learning, but the mind is strong and powerful; some noted scholars

▶ *Rocine: "You have few, if any, negative personality aspects! You have untapped genius!"*

- Gourmet tastes
- Are slow to forgive
- Lack self-confidence
- Your humility is genuine
- Love nature and the outdoors
- Some have an addictive tendency
- Born philosophers and naturalists
- Feelings are strong and controlled
- Need time alone within a relationship
- Love God, the universe, a higher power
- Appear meek and powerless, but are not!
- Have faith, hope, and courage (no suicides)
- Have a reserved nature (unlike other Fat types)
- Sexual drive slight to medium and rarely a priority
- Males are home-bodies: love cooking, gardening, etc.
- Have low self-confidence (high willpower if motivated)
- Are careful with all actions; rarely seek fame and fortune
- Mind is slow but very efficient (difficult to take examinations)
- Generally ignore rudeness, intolerance or sarcasm from others

- Respect people who work hard; have no time for the homeless
- Have strong likes, and strong dislikes that are hard to overcome
- Display peace, interest, friendliness, concern, and interest in others
- Are loyal, law abiding, hard working, ethical, vigilant supervisors: employers benefit from hiring you

▶ *You are plain, friendly, high-minded, and practical; you learn from life. You do the right thing. You are trustful and talk heart-to-heart with anyone.*

———

Barotic Potential Challenges

You may have evolved from or not experienced these general challenges, so do not dwell on them.

- Make poor investors
- Need time before taking action
- Tend to over-indulge in the senses
- Low self-confidence hampers accomplishments
- May be shy, reticent, suspicious, self-depreciating

- May lack judgment in selecting mates and employees
- Are "slow to ripen;" rarely feel appreciated when young
- Are somewhat intolerant of moral improprieties of others
- If pushed to your limit, you explode with pent-up emotions
- May feel disadvantaged in society due to plain speech and dress
- Intensely dislike laziness, vanity, crime, ugliness, chaos, disorder
- Upset by wrong conduct in others, but try to be non-judgmental
- If severely wronged, that person can do nothing right; you look for redress and may lose control of your tongue

▶ *If you relate to any of these challenges, doing something to overcome them serves your evolution.*

Stress Management

You have strong *mental* stress prevention giving you good resistance to internalizing this stress into your stomach, adrenals, and immune system. *Emotional* stress prevention is also strong, a tribute to your balanced mind.

[If needing help managing these stresses, see my prior books.]

Love

You are romantic, faithful and often attracted to the *atrophic, sillevitic, pathoferic, myogenic, nervimotive, and neurogenic* types. Before marriage, you usually become a life-long friend of your mate.

———

Talents and Vocations

Abilities — *Human communications, executives, outdoor activities, management, service, restaurant, and food professions*

You are highly practical and able to apply principles, laws, facts, or theories and make them work. Employers prize your honesty and work-ethic. You are good judges of art, and usually not highly educated; but occasionally you are great scholars. You love nature.

▶ *I have known or observed you as gardeners, managers, chemists, photographers, leasing agents, home-makers; a minister, musician, scientist, doctor, homeless man, and real estate and stock market brokers. One man, a Ph.D. in literature, was a highly acclaimed book critic for a major U.S. newspaper—a very humble man, unlike most fat types!*

The type information cannot predict what or whom you will become, but you are capable of bringing a creative excellence or brilliance to whatever you do in life.

Inabilities — *Indoor work, temperature extremes*

You rarely self-actualize or own your own business, preferring instead to serve others. You are happiest working outdoors, and although capable of learning, are not attracted to law, medicine, or intense study.

▶ *Rocine: "Barotic skills are not in the fingers or hands, but are in your brain and mind. Even so, you rarely achieve anything before age 50-60."*

Health Problems

You are usually quite healthy until later in life, but when sick you commonly experience health problems or diseases in the following areas:

Circulation — Your circulatory system is particularly weak and susceptible to fatty diseases.

Heart — A poor diet, lack of exercise, and obesity affect your heart: you may need medication.

Gout and Arthritis — Your usual acid-ash diet (excess meat and carbohydrates) promotes joint disease, arthritis, or gout.

———

Barotic Acid/Alkaline Factor

[See Chapter 3 for details on this subject, along with the common symptoms found with people of different nervous system dominance.]

For your health and healing, your nervous system genetics require a specific ratio of acid to alkaline foods. You are born with **intermediate** dominance (between *para-sympathetic* and *sympathetic*), and need *balanced* acid and alkaline-ash food intake. (Ash refers to the minerals left in your body after metabolizing foods.) You may indulge in both food classes. Construct this approximate ratio of food selections:

50% Fruits, salads, vegetables
50% Proteins, carbohydrates

▶ *Approximate your food ratios. On any particular day, it does not matter if one meal is mostly alkaline and another mostly acid—just try to balance it out for the day! If you make a mistake, try again tomorrow. It is a subjective call that you make, and what is done over time that makes the difference to your health.*

_____

Barotic Spiritual Factor

Skip this paragraph if uninterested in a type philosophical perspective!

▶ *Rocine: "The soul chooses the body type."*

If as souls, we choose the brain and body type to spend a lifetime in, it could be to learn certain spiritual lessons related to perfecting ourselves, and our humanity, in God's eyes. What lessons does the type bring you? Only you can really decide what those lessons are. You know your weaknesses, faults, and behaviors towards others. You know things about yourself that Victor Rocine could never get from his research subjects when he first wrote about types. So search your mind for the answers.

Each discrete type has challenges of life lessons, spiritual goals, etc., and some of yours may be:

Faith — Your faith, based in nature and natural law, is in the goodness of man (you are deeply hurt when this premise proves wrong).

Fat — Your fat is genetic, but weight can be lost so work on it, or fat-related cardio-vascular diseases are likely.

Non-judgmental — You sit on the fence on important issues, and do not judge others; sometimes a judgment needs to be made!

———

A Barotic Story...

William, age 44, 5'7, 340 pounds, fatigued, and listless, took medication for heart problems. Examination showed dietary excesses of carbon and hydrogen foods: carbohydrates, syrups, proteins (meat, poultry, fish, cheese), starches, grains, breads, sweet fruits, and alcohol.

He also showed deficits in sodium and trace mineral foods: scallops, lobster, fish, milk, cheese, kelp, olives, raw cabbage, Swiss chard, beet greens, celery, and cod liver oil.

He made these dietary changes, took the herbs indicated for his type, and soon made good progress.

———

Barotic Type Mineral Foods

Apply this mineral data to the diet following the Fat type descriptions.

Excessive Foods:

- *Calcium*
- *Carbon (simple carbohydrates)*
- *Nitrogen (beef)*
- *Sulfur (cooked)*
- *Sodium (salted, junk)*

Deficient Foods:

- *Trace Minerals*
- *Nitrogen (non-beef, vegetable)*
- *Sulfur (raw)*
- *Sodium (unsalted, non-junk)*

These deficient nutrients are common deficiencies in your type, and predispose you to ill-health. If ill, be sure to use these lists with your daily food intake. If not ill, eat from the food lists 3-4 days weekly for maintenance. All food lists are in descending order of concentration and value to you; choose servings of foods in the upper half of each list first!
One serving is ½ cup.

Barotic Excessive Foods -

Calcium is excessively absorbed in your tissues. It is highly concentrated in your bones, joints, muscles, nerves, heart, teeth, and gums; if you have an illness or disease in any of these tissues decreasing calcium foods and supplements may be a significant healing factor.

Carbon is excessive in your type, so minimize it. It is excessive in all people who become fat or obese and is in every cell of the body as the basis of life.

Nitrogen from red meat is excessive in your diet (if eaten more than twice monthly), and is a major cause of your acidity and illnesses; eat poultry, fish and eggs about 3-4 days weekly with vegetarian proteins like legumes (peas, beans), seeds, nuts and pasta on the other days.

Sulfur is excessive in cooked foods, producing excessive sulfur acid toxicity—raw sulfur foods preclude this happening.

Sodium from salted junk foods is excessive in your tissues. To preserve your health and weight control you should avoid junk foods and fulfill your sodium needs from the food list (without the salt-shaker).

_____

Deficient foods -

In illness or disease, it is important to correct these deficiencies.

Trace minerals may become deficient in your type.

Nitrogen from vegetable sources is deficient (see above note).

Sulfur from raw food sources is deficient in your tissues. It is important for body detoxifying.

Sodium from non-salted foods is deficient in your type (see above note).

[See the Appendix for descriptive notes on minerals.]

_____

[The following recommendations are for the generic type. Additionally, you may need from a holistic healer or nutritionist, something more specific for your individuality.]

Minimize
Excessive Foods

Calcium: *1-2 servings/week only*
Swiss and cheddar cheese, turnip greens, almonds, brewer's yeast, parsley, corn tortillas, dandelion greens, brazil nuts, watercress, tofu.

Carbon: *1-2 servings/week only*
***Avoid* simple** *carbohydrates: white and brown sugars, high fructose corn syrup, honey, maple syrup, molasses, jellies, candy, ice cream, soda drinks.*
***Eat* complex** *carbohydrates: yams, potatoes, squash, pumpkin, corn, lentils, peas, beans, green vegetables, grains.*

Nitrogen (animal): *0-1 times/month*
Beef, red meats

Sulfur (cooked): *1-2 servings/week only*
Cabbage, onions, cauliflower, garlic, Brussels sprouts, broccoli, turnips, mustard greens, rutabagas

Minimize…

> ### **Sodium (salted, junk):**
> *1-2 servings/week only*
> *Salt, all fast foods, packaged foods, canned and frozen foods, preserved meats (cured, smoked, canned), sauces (soy, barbecue, catsup, etc.), pizza, chips (potato, corn, etc.), dill pickles, sauerkraut, bouillon cubes, peanut butter, salted nuts, crackers, canned or packaged soups, processed cheeses, commercial salad dressings.*
> *Note: If you should eat anything on this list, keep it down to ½ cup weekly!*

Eat
Deficient Foods

Trace Minerals: *1-2 servings/day*

Kelp, goat's cheese and milk, raw garlic, sprouts, rhubarb, beet greens, peach, alfalfa, ginger, rice, oats, pineapples, dry split peas, blackstrap molasses, seeds, nuts, brown rice, oat straw and alfalfa teas.

Nitrogen (non-beef, vegetable):

Black-eyed peas, beans, lentils, seeds, spirulina — as desired
Eggs, poultry, fish — 3-5 times weekly

Sulfur (raw): *1-2 servings/day*

Cauliflower, cabbage, onions, spinach, figs, carrots, horseradish, radishes, chestnuts, egg whites, oranges, shrimp

Sodium (unsalted, non-junk):
1-2 servings/day

Olives, kelp, celery (and juice), lentils, almonds, cheese (Roquefort, cottage, Swiss), Swiss chard, beets and greens, okra, pistachio, sesame seeds, turnips, carrots, yogurt, strawberry, oatmeal.

Barotic Nutritional Supplements

- **Multi-Vitamins** —
  [Take all supplements with food.]
  2 capsules/day with food
- **Do not take Calcium or Multi-Minerals** —
  You already have excessive calcium in your body (Exception: menopausal, on estrogen, osteoporosis)
- **Kelp** —
  6 tablets/once daily with food.
- **Herbs** —
  Brain detox – Ginkgo or Gotu Kola
  Organ detox – Milk Thistle or
  Strawberry Leaf
  (Take one capsule, twice daily; then one, three times weekly)
- **Evening Primrose or Flaxseed Oil** —
  1 soft-gel/day with food
- **Other** —
  Chlorophyll, blue-green algae, green magma, spirulina, alfalfa, or other source
  (Take as directed: take one, three times weekly.)

Important Barotic Health Concerns

Your nervous system genetics require the *Fat* type Food Guide for health, and any carnivorous cravings are normal and healthy for you. After age 50, however, you need flesh only three days weekly.

If vegetarian, make sure you eat enough vegetable proteins daily (and in addition to food protein, you usually require a protein drink of 25-30 gm., 3-4 days weekly).

Instead of diet pills, you need glucomanin supplements that prevent over-eating by swelling and taking up space in the stomach!

BAROTIC FOOD GUIDE

Aim for –
50% Proteins, carbohydrates
50% Fruits, salads, vegetables
and
50% Raw food diet
50% Cooked foods
Stop eating beef!
Lose the salt shaker.
Take the recommended supplements.

▶ *Rocine: "Under great stress you become great. In times of peace and plenty, you are a sleeping genius."*

––––––

Barotic Weight Loss

Losing weight depends upon you following the type instructions, summarized in this section (see list).

- *Stop* eating simple carbohydrates and sodium foods (see list)
- *Protein* drink daily, about 25-30 grams
- *Eat* your body type deficient mineral foods daily
- *Follow* your *Barotic Guide (as above)*
- *Exercise*: your body type requires light to moderate daily exercise (like yoga, walking)
- *Simple sugars*: stop all white table sugar and high-fructose corn syrup and drinks containing these sugars
- *Calories:* As with any dietary approach, calories in, must be *less than* calories out! Most markets sell a calorie booklet; make notes of your daily intake, and in most instances keep it under about 1500-1800 calories/day

––––––

Fat Types
General Food Guide

(Intermediate between Carnivores and strict Vegetarian)

Important Note

―――――

The Food Guide addresses the <u>Acid-Alkaline</u> aspect of your food intake, along with the <u>Type Mineral</u> factor presented throughout this book. It does <u>not</u> necessarily address calories or other dietary factors that may be pertinent to your personal health needs whether medical or appropriate for some other dietary need. So use your common sense and just include the factors described here with whatever healthy dietary choices you usually make.

For other nutrient information, consult with nutritional books or with holistic nutritional doctors. In this regard, I particularly recommend the advice of Andrew Weil, M.D.

―――――

Fat Types
General Food Guide

This chapter presents an <u>Intermediate</u> Food Guide, balanced between the Muscle types (carnivores) and the Thin types (vegetarians). Superimpose the individual type mineral and other information from your type chapter into this Food Guide (which is not for the pargenic type.)

———

Meat/Flesh Intake

Generally, animal protein is acceptable and needed in your diet: red meat should be limited to once weekly or less, while lamb and fish or poultry are excellent in moderation. If this diet is similar to what you are already eating, but you have health problems because of a history of excess acid-ash food intake being so common, then:

- Decrease your carbohydrate and protein intake by about one-third
- Increase your fruit, salad and vegetable intake by about one-third
- Consult with a holistic doctor, preferably one versed in nutritional and emotional evaluation

———

Over-Acid or Over-Alkaline?

Just as a log of wood burned in your fireplace leaves a mineral-ash, food ash refers to the minerals remaining after metabolizing foods in your tissues:

- Fruits and vegetables **alkalinize** tissues
- Proteins and carbohydrates **acidify** tissues

You are usually over-acid due to:

- Accumulated metabolic waste-acids
- Deficient fruit, salad and vegetable intake
- Excessive protein and carbohydrate intake

You need to estimate the ratio of foods being eaten. Generally, eat the following *approximate* ratio of foods for your health:

> 50% *Alkaline-ash* foods (fruits, salads, vegetables)
> 50% *Acid-ash* foods (complex carbohydrates like starches, grains, cereals, breads, flour products; and proteins)

Approximate your food ratios. On any particular day it does not matter if one meal is mostly alkaline, and another is acid—just try to balance it out for the day! If you make a mistake, forget it and try again tomorrow. It is a subjective call that you make. It is what you do over weeks and months that makes the difference to your health—not on any few days.

The net result is that the Fat types require the plan presented in this chapter for health restoration.

[The following chart shows the fat types, their acid-alkaline reactions, and the percentage of raw foods needed for their healing.]

Fat Types

Acid/Alkaline Genetics
Dietary-Ash and Raw Food Needs

———

This chart shows the Rocine types, their acid or alkaline food needs, and the percentage of raw foods needed for your health and healing.

BODY TYPE	ACID/ALKALINE GENETICS	% DIETARY ASH	% RAW FOODS
Barotic	Intermediate	50:50	50
Carboferic	Intermediate	50:50	50
Hydripheric	Intermediate	50:50	30
Isogenic	Intermediate	50:50	30
Lipopheric	Intermediate	50:50	50
Oxypheric	Intermediate	50:50	50
Pargenic	Acid	70% alkaline	30

Note that the above percentages will vary depending on aging and the health of individual types.

Notes

- Never eat foods you are allergic to, no matter what I recommend here; if you suspect allergy to a suggested food, eliminate it.
- Minimize your white sugar and alcohol intake.
- Eat the right foods most of the time and the diet will help you; you do not have to live out of a health food store (although such foods are healthier).
- All food lists are in descending order of concentration and value to you as a mineral source; whenever possible, choose foods in the upper half of each list first! One serving is ½ cup.
- If desired, you may interchange lunches for dinners.
- Avoid all junk foods, white sugar, foods with added sugar, and high fructose corn syrup

———

Fat Types / General Food Guide

Breakfasts

[Superimpose the nutritional information from your Type Chapter into this Food Guide.]

EGGS (1-2) with lettuce, tomato, whole grain toast — 1-3 times/week; or

FRUIT SALAD, fresh with citrus fruit and a protein source (low-sugar yogurt, kefir, milk, cottage cheese, cheese, seeds or nuts) — 2-4 times/week; or

COOKED CEREALS, fruit, seeds, whole grain, and nuts — 2-5 times/week; or

OTHER — 0-1 times/week

Eat unlimited fruit, salads, vegetables, with seeds/nuts for snacks. Wheat is a common allergy: avoid white and wheat breads

* * *

DAILY LIQUIDS

Pure water — as desired (except Hydripheric type) Fruit and vegetable juices — 0-2 cups Coffee, caffeine teas — 0-2 cups
[Include selections from your type mineral needs with each meal.]

Lunches

SALADS, mixed green, and 2-4 oz., of protein (fish, poultry, egg, cheese, tofu, seeds or nuts, etc.). [Dressings: use canola or olive oil* and vinegar; or low-fat/calorie dressing]
— 2-4 times/week; or

VEGETABLES (steamed) with salad, and yogurt, or cottage cheese (or other breakfast proteins) — 1-2 times/week; or

FRUIT SALAD (see breakfast)
— 0-1 times/week

SANDWICH, whole grains with a non-flesh protein (egg, tofu, cheese, etc.)
—1-3 times/week; or

POULTRY, FISH, 3-4 oz., with a mixed green salad and/or steamed vegetables (or as a sandwich) —1-2 times/week; or

OTHER — 0-1 times/week

* Other oils less ideal; soybean is common allergen; minimize commercial dressings

[Include selections from your type mineral needs with each meal.]

Dinners

LEAN POULTRY OR FISH *(4-6 oz.)*
— 2-4 times/week

PASTA, PROTEIN *(as above)*
—1-3 times/week

VEGETARIAN MEAL, *including legumes,
tofu, cheese, cottagecheese, seeds or nuts, egg, etc.*
—2-4 times/week

LEAN BEEF *(4-6 oz.)*
— 0-2 times/month

OTHER *— 0-2 times/week*

*Take all of the above with: mixed green salad,
dressing (as before), and/or vegetables.*

DESSERTS
Fruits, fresh — as desired
Low-sugar, healthy desserts —0-3 times/week

*If you have blood fat problems, cholesterol or
triglycerides, eliminate all beef from your diet,
and see my earlier books. Eat fruit, unlimited
salads and vegetables with seeds/nuts, low-sugar
yogurt for snacks.*

**[Include selections from your type mineral
needs with each meal.]**

Fat Types Notes

Do not eat flesh everyday: have it on alternate days only. For munchies, have low calorie items like celery and other vegetables, along with yogurt and cottage cheese, etc. Some of you abuse your beef and red meat intake, perhaps several times weekly—this is a false craving; use your will to combat it if you want to be healthier!

Steamed Vegetables — Minerals are lost in the boiling of vegetables; best is steaming or wok cooking.

Minimize Foods — Only eat them 0-1 times/week! Be sure to eat the recommended foods to help your healing;

Food Combinations —Eating proteins at the same meal with starches often results in indigestion, gas or constipation (along with low blood sugar and making fat). Watch how this inharmonious food combination may be affecting you.

Minimize —
- All fatty foods
- Milk and dairy foods (unless otherwise noted)
- Commercial, sugared, and fatty salad dressings

- Beef, sugar, wines, alcohol, coffee, white sugar, red meats, and processed meats

Vegetarian Proteins — If you choose to be vegetarian, it will help your health after middle-age; because you have semi-carnivorous genes be sure to take a protein supplement of 20-30 grams/day (e.g., soy or egg-white powder in juice).

Healthy Weight — Invariably you hold excessive weight, and in addition to body type factors there may be a medical problem behind your fat storage. By eating according to your body type, you slowly and naturally lose excess weight! Accumulating evidence indicts high-fructose corn syrup as a major cause of increased weight and obesity. Avoid it!

You have a sluggish fat-burning metabolism, and may have an under-active adrenal, thyroid, or pituitary gland resulting in hypoglycemia, and in this instance may need the services of a holistic doctor *(see Appendix* and my earlier books).

———

In Conclusion

I hope you have enjoyed reading this book. You should now know your body type and have learned some valuable information about how to be a healthier you! Do not forget the my previous books on healing yourself.

If you desire further help or information with your body type or health from a holistic viewpoint, email me from page one of my web page: Dr.Stenbeck.net

Good health and good luck!

———

Appendix

Brief Extracts from
<u>The 22 Unique Body Types</u>

Appendix A

Types
(Brief extract)

Type comes from 'typus' meaning an image or impression, the study of types being called typology.

▶ *Rocine: "A combination of mental and structural features is consistently found in people of the same type."*

Rocine wrote that all types are a mixture of positive and negative qualities. He based his work on the biochemical individuality of our *mineral* absorption and utilization. Of course, all minerals are absorbed, but he postulated that different types of people *selectively* absorb certain minerals, to a greater or lesser extent, requiring specific mineral foods for their enhanced health and healing.

▶ *The type information cannot predict what or who you will become, or how successful or not, but your type is capable of bringing a creative excellence to whatever you do in life. If your type has negative qualities that you disagree with, remember that they are only tendencies and may or may not manifest in you.*

This book enlarges on Rocine's premise (early 1900's), integrated with the later research of Herbert Sheldon, M.D., Ph.D., at Harvard University (1930's), along with my fifty years of observations and experience with this subject.

Comparing your shared physical (and sometimes psychological) descriptions with the Celebrity Lists further assists the identification of your type. It is not that you will look exactly like, or be a twin to, any particular celebrity. Look closely at a celebrity's features: face, profile, height, weight, head, etc. If you know something about their talents, beliefs, success and failure spheres, health and weight challenges, attitudes and behaviors, etc., then you get clues as to what your type may be.

―――――

Understanding Types and Sub-Types

Each of us has a clearly discernible dominant type. Visualize the celebrity examples from movies, politics, sports, the arts and public life, and try to identify with their physical features. Look for similar features, remembering that you will not recognize all attributes in yourself. You are not looking for your twin!

The sub-type issue is the main reason people of the same major type can look so different. Remember that a type description does not characterize you exactly, but depicts your individual variant of a type.

▶ *The type questionnaire pinpoints the major features of that type: if the celebrity examples are unhelpful, you may be an unusual variant (in which case ignore the celebrity issue and give yourself 7 points on Question 1).*

———

Minerals

Minerals are essential life nutrients that accelerate enzyme and chemical reactions and provide a basis for your body typing. Although found in all tissues, different minerals tend to be concentrated in certain organs, their presence or absence contributing to the healing of such tissues; e.g., zinc accelerates prostate healing; calcium and manganese promote bone, joint and connective tissue healing.

Specific foods nurture each type, some people needing meats for their health others needing a vegetarian diet. A high potassium diet nurtures one person, while another needs high sulfur, calcium, zinc, or another mineral.

Mineral Digestion and Absorption

Compared to vitamins, minerals are *difficult* to digest, absorb, and utilize. In people with strong digestive systems, this aspect may not be important. The following factors should be in place for optimal mineral metabolism:

1. Stomach Hydrochloric Acid Production
2. Parathyroid Hormone Balance
3. Organ Toxic Metal and Chemical Removal
   [See details in <u>The 22 Unique Body Types</u>.*]*

———

Total Body Healing

Note that from a holistic healing perspective, in addition to minerals and type information, the following healing factors are necessary:

Nutrient Balance
Mental Balance
Emotional Balance
Spiritual Balance
Detoxifying Integrity

The above factors are all important to your total healing especially if you are interested in self-healing (see my earlier books).

———

Appendix B

Researchers
(Brief extract)

The predominant workers in this area of human individuality from around 1880's to the 1960's are Herbert Sheldon, M.D., Ph.D., Roger Williams, Ph.D., and Victor Rocine, D.Sc.

Much information on Sheldon's research exists on-line and in medical psychology libraries; for interested readers there are other lines of research published in the last century. This present book is primarily about Rocine's body types.

Herbert Sheldon M.D., Ph.D.

In contrast to Rocine, Sheldon at Harvard University in the 1930's was trained in the scientific method and did painstaking research and publishing on human individuality. In comparing his findings with Rocine's work, a direct putative correlation is visible.

Roger J. Williams, Ph.D.

Another significant researcher in human individuality is the renowned scientist and biochemist, Roger J. Williams. He demonstrated that different people have varying levels of nutrients, enzymes, and other metabolic chemicals in their bloodstreams.

▶ *Williams's research firmly expands on the premise of individual nutritional needs in human beings. If interested in his research, I highly recommend his book Biochemial Individuality.*

Victor Rocine, D.Sc.

Note that when a negative feature is indicated, say neurotic tendencies, all members of the type are <u>not</u> that way; it is a type tendency reported by Rocine.

Rocine studied type-related diseases finding links between mineral and dietary factors with individual types and their diseases. In each body type, one or more dominant minerals are preferentially absorbed and utilized over other minerals.

He recognized discrete body types from their physical appearance finding genetically based mineral dominance to be the determining feature. He also correlated their physical features with psychological characteristics.

——

Genetics, Types, and Diet
(Brief extract)

This section deals with how nervous system genetics helps determine your eating choices for health: you are either born to be a predominant meat eater, a partial or complete vegetarian, or something between the two. The genetic factor determining this dietary aspect is the *sympathetic and parasympathetic* components of your central nervous system. This represents a basic factor in eating for health.

This chapter helps you understand your dietary inheritance, although instinctively, you may already have arrived there!

- If born **sympathetic** dominant you are *genetically acid*, desiring a predominantly *vegetarian* diet for your health (about 70% fruit, salad, vegetables to 30% proteins and carbohydrates).

- If born **parasympathetic** dominant you are *genetically alkaline*, desiring a predominantly *carnivorous* diet for your health (about 70% proteins, carbohydrates to 30% fruits, salads, vegetables). Few of you ever choose to become vegetarian because of the difficulty in satisfying your protein needs without meats.

- If born ***intermediate*** dominant you
  may eat food groups with little concern
  for the acid/alkaline factor. However,
  after age 40, you need a semi-vegetarian
  diet for healthy eating.

———

Chart of Relative Nervous System Dominance

In the following Chart, if you relate to many
of the symptoms on one side you probably
have that nervous system dominance; relating
to both sides indicates *Intermediate* dominance.

If Vegetarian (Over-acid) --
  Eat 70% fruits, salads, vegetables
  And 30% proteins, carbohydrates

If Carnivore (Over-alkaline) --
  Eat 70% proteins, carbohydrates
  And 30% fruits, salads, vegetables

If Intermediate --
  Eat 50:50 of acid and alkaline-ash foods

Make an *approximate* estimate of your daily
acid and alkaline food intake (such ratios varying
from type to type).

———

Symptoms of Relative Genetic Dominance

Vegetarians (Over-acid)	Carnivores (Over-alkaline)
Sympathetic Dominance	*Parasympathetic Dominance*
little or no flesh desire	*desire flesh*
easily constipated	*rarely constipated*
slow digestion	*fast digestion*
easily dehydrated	*not dehydrated*
strong thirst	*low thirst*
pale face	*flushed face*
high pulse after food	*slow pulse after food*
easy gag reflex	*slow gag reflex*
cool dry skin	*moist warm skin*
nervous stomach	*calm stomach*
little eyelid blinking	*much blinking*
nervous tendency	*mostly calm*
slower healing	*faster healing*
low oxygen-uptake	*good oxygen-uptake*
easily breathless	*seldom breathless*
insomnia common	*sleep easier*
few muscle cramps	*some night cramps*
calcium deposits rare	*get calcium deposits*

Appendix D

Help Identifying your Body Type with Dr. Stenbeck

If you desire help in identifying your body type, follow these instructions, and answer the questionnaire. For further information and fees, send me an email from page one of the website:

DrStenbeck.net

First name: _____

Country of birth: _____

Upload photos and send to the above website:

- Head and shoulders: front and side views

- Full body: front and side views

- Also 1-2 teenage views

- If possible, casual photos of mother, father, siblings

MY TYPE CLASS MAY BE: _____

   (Thin, Muscle, or Fat)

AGE   -   _____

HEIGHT   -   _____ feet/inches

MY WEIGHT -   _____ pounds

   Heaviest at age: _____

- Lightest as adult: _____

- Estimate age 15: _____

VISION - Excellent Average   Poor:

HAIR - Natural color: _____

   - Thin/thick?   _____

   - balding?   _____

SKIN - Quality: _____

   - History of acne, boils, other:

_____

_____

TEETH   - Strong   Weak   Dentures

      - Cavity history: Many   Moderate   Few

MUSCLES - Strong   Average   Weak

    Sports played _____

JOINTS   - Strong   Average   Weak

HEALTH - Childhood diseases?

_____

_____

- Adult diseases?

_____

AVERAGE DIET

- Beef _____ (times/week)

 - Poultry _____ (times/week)

 - Fish _____ (times/week)

 - Eggs _____ (times/week)

 - Water _____ (glasses/day):

 - Vegetarian? Vegan? _____

 - Other? _____

 - Did your childhood diet differ? _____

The above will help me know who you are! I will send you a follow-up questionnaire for further help in identifying your body type.

Appendix E

On-line Health Consultation with Dr. Stenbeck

For further information, or to comment on this book, or to receive a response on any health issue from a holistic viewpoint, send an email inquiry from page one of my website:

DrStenbeck.net

Following that, I will suggest further healing needs, which we may pursue with an on-line consult.

———

Appendix F

Notes

See my book *The 22 Unique Body Types,* available at the usual online source, for further information and details on all of the 22 Types. The Appendix in that book has further information about:

Mineral Functions and Food Sources

Further Reading

———